I0435327

Compliance

And Living a Good Life

Living with a Coumadin, low sodium,

restricted liquids, and diabetic diets.

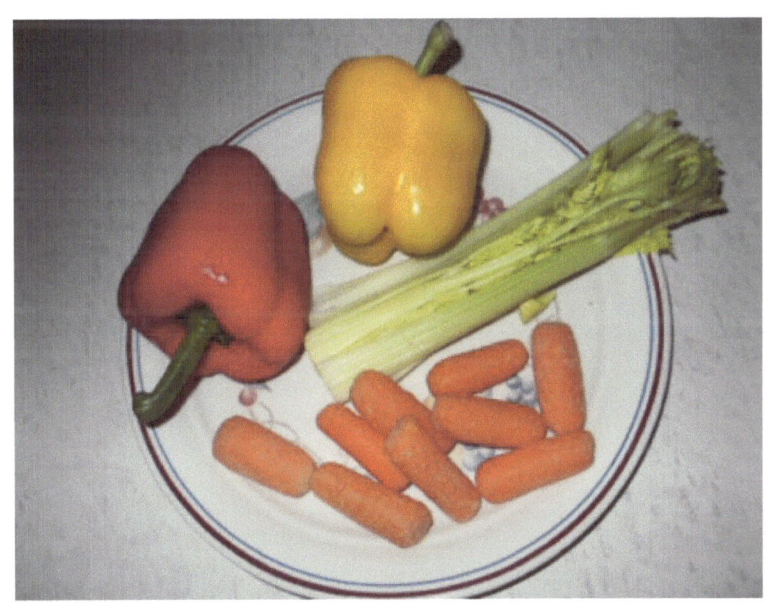

How I handled and coped with

a total lifestyle change

Bennie F. Wingate- Author

Mildred E. Hamilton-Editor

Contents

All rights reserved. All text are copyrighted material. No portion of this book may be reproduced except charts and recipes. Library of Congress Cataloging –in-Publication Data

Bennie F. Wingate- Author

bennie_wingate@yahoo.com

Mildred E. Hamilton- Editor

queenofthesth@att.net

Copyright 2014

Brief History of how it all started

On the morning of 17 September 2013 I was rushed to the emergency room at local hospital. When I came to It, had been determined that I had Atrial Fibrillation. I stayed in the hospital for 6 days. While I was in the hospital I was also informed that I also had diabetes. This added on another issue along with the heart issue.

During my stay the hospital, the dietitians briefed me on all the do's and don'ts of my conditions. Believe me it was a lot of don't and very little do's. So I collected all the information pamphlets that they had. The hospital was very helpful and willing to work with me on changing my eating habits and my lifestyle.

At that time I worked 3rd shift on a great job at a product plant. At my own doing I had very bad sleep habits, like sleeping in short spells and not getting enough sleep. While all this was going on I had very bad eating habits. I was eating almost all fast food and at the wrong times. Eating just before going to bed was the norm. I was eating all kind of fried foods and junk foods, without worrying about the sodium, sugar, fats.

 All that added up to a brick wall with a serious medical condition. I hit that wall real hard and almost did not make it. After a long conference with my heart doctor, my son and sister I decided to make a complete change in my total lifestyle.

 It has been about 6 months now and I am doing very well. My Heart is under control and working very well. The diabetes is under control with very little medicines. I have trimmed down by 40 pounds and feel better than I have felt in over five years. The doctors and nurses say that I am one of the most compliant patents they have ever seen.

I am writing this as a guide so as to help others with these issues. I hope that they can use the information to have a better, longer and healthier lifestyle.

First Days home

I will be the first to admit that I was nervous the first days at home. While I was in the hospital all I could think about was going home. While I was in the hospital I had gotten used to being surrounded by medical personal. When I got home I realized that the medical staff was gone, an it was up to me to follow the guide lines laid out by the doctors and nurses. I was very blessed to have a son and sister that were there for any and every thing that I needed. My son that the time was going to nursing school and my sister lives right next door which both combined was a winning combination.

Besides all the physical changes and adjustments I had to have a mental change of lifestyle also. Before any physical change could be conquered I had to mentally make up my mind to live right and follow all the guidelines given to me. The hospital provided my with a lot of information I needed, but it was up to me to make it happen. The biggest change was going to be my very unhealthy eating habits.

Here is a basic list of the restrictions.

1. Low vitamin K due to taking Coumadin
2. Low sodium, less than 2000mg day
3. Restricted liquids, less that 2 liters a day
4. Diabetic diet using less sugars
5. No Beef

This became a shopping challenge at first. With all the restrictions we had to read every label of everything we bought. After the second trip to the grocery store I made a list of everything we bought with the sodium, sugars, cholesterol, Vitamin K, and calories content. After doing that It became real easy to shop and stay within the guidelines I needed for healthy eating.

Change of lifestyle and eating habits

Lifestyle

The lifestyle was the easiest part to make a change. That was just a matter of getting plenty of rest on a good schedule. Changing things around so as not to let stress but a part of my life. Having a low impact daily exercise program, mainly consisting of walking as tolerated. All walking is under Guidance of a doctor and done with common sense.

Eating Habits

The eating habits were the biggest and most challenging change that we had to adapt to. Cutting out the fast food restaurants was relatively easily. Stopping the use of beef was not a problem either. Not using processed meats was a big challenge because we were using them almost all the time. This is things like hotdogs, sliced lunch meats, canned hams, processed hams, TV dinners, the list goes on and on. All of the foods that we ate everyday were on that list.

The first thing we changed was buying only fresh meats or frozen fresh meats. This included chicken, turkey, pork, fish and wild game but no beef. Canned vegetables have a lot of sodium so we started getting fresh or fresh frozen vegetables only. Just about all fresh or fresh frozen vegetables have no or very low sodium.

Having to take Coumadin also means that I had to reduce the intake of vitamin K. Vitamin K counteracts the coumadin and the more Vitamin K, the more coumadin it takes the adjust to the correct level. This took out all the leafy vegetables plus a lot of other vegetables. Vitamin K is not listed on the Nutrition Facts label thus making it had to track. There is a list of Foods with Vitamin K in the pamphlet to help when buying foods.

The biggest help came from my son and my sister. My son eats whatever I cook for me that make meal planning very easy. When my sister comes over to eat her and her husband eat the same things that I eat. The family was the biggest support of all.

Tips for tracking liquids and food contents

The best way that I found to track the liquid is to use a marked container. Take a plastic container and put a piece of tape at the level of the maximum intake you can have in a day. Mark it with a color that you can see real well. You can measure it out each time you have something to drink and write it down on a piece of paper to keep track of it. I found that the easiest way was to do this and just pour the liquid into the container and you can see how much you have consumed and how much more you can have.

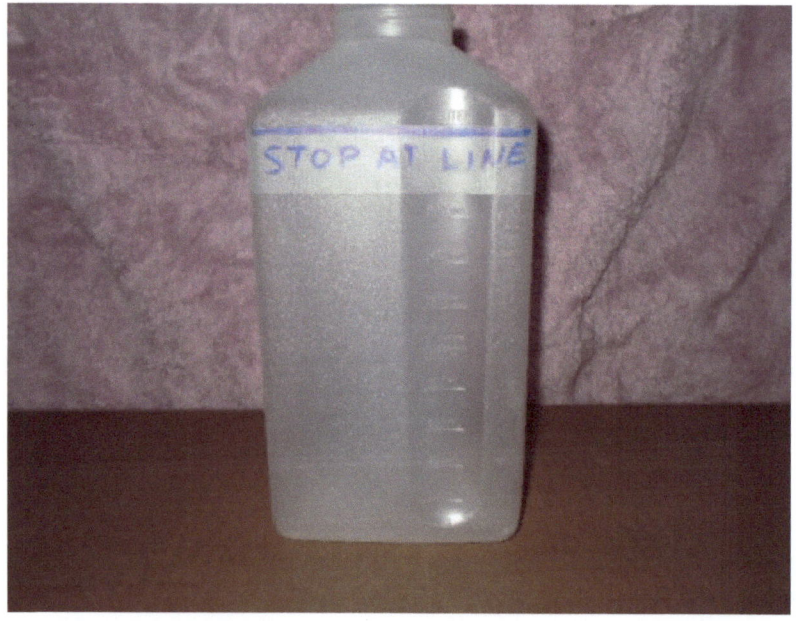

Helpful ways of tracking Dietary needs

There are blank charts in the back of this pamphlet that we created. By using these charts I was able to shop and buy the healthiest foods. All the blank charts in the back can be reproduced for you conveyance. They also helped me control intake of foods that kept me within the doctors guide lines.

Vitamin K is not listed on The Nutrition Facts label that is displayed on foods. To a person taking Coumadin, Vitamin K is a very important part on that diet. Here is a chart that helps you find foods that will fit into your dietary needs.

High Vitamin K (more than 100mcg)

Food	Serving	mcg
Broccoli	½ cup	110
Brussels sprouts	½ cup	109
Endive, raw	1 cup	116
Greens, beet	½ cup	350
Greens, collard, frozen	½ cup	530
Greens, turnip	½ cup	265
Greens, turnip, frozen	½ cup	425
Kale, fresh, or frozen	½ cup	531
Kale, raw	½ cup	274
Onions, green or scallion	½ cup	105
Parsley	10 sprigs	164
Spinach	½ cup	444
Spinach, raw	1 cup	145
Swiss chard	½ cup	287

Moderate Vitamin K (25-100 mcg)

Food	Serving	mcg
Asparagus	5 spears	38
Asparagus, frozen	½ cup	72
Broccoli, raw	½ cup	45
Food	Serving	mcg
Cabbage	½ cup	37
Cabbage, green	½ cup	82
Dried peas, blackeye	½ cup	32
Kiwi fruit	1 medium	31
Lettuce, green leaf	1 cup	63
Lettuce, romaine	1 cup	57
Noodles, spinach	½ cup	81

Food	Serving	mcg
Okra, frozen	½ cup	44
Prunes, dried	5 each	25
Watercress, raw	1 cup	85

Low Vitamin K (less than25 mcg)

Food	Serving	mcg
Artichoke	1 medium	18
Avocado, raw	1 oz	6
Beans, green or yellow	½ cup	10
Blackberries or blueberries	½ cup	14
Cabbage, raw	½ cup	21
Carrots	½ cup	11
Cauliflower, raw	½ cup	8
Celery, raw	½ cup	18
Cucumber, with peel	½ cup	9
Food	**Serving**	**mcg**
Dried beans and peas, most types	½ cup	5-9
Grapes	½ cup	12
Lettuce, iceberg	1 cup	13
Mango	1 medium	9
Margarine-blend, tub or stick	1 tbsp.	13-15
Mayonnaise	1 tbsp.	6
Nuts, pine, cashews	1 oz	15
Oil, olive	1 tbsp.	8
Oils, such as soybean, canola, salad	1 tbsp.	10-25
Papaya	1 medium	8
Parsley, dried	1 tbsp.	18
Pear	1 medium	8
Peas, green	½ cup	19
Pickles, dill or kosher	1 spear	14
Salad dressings	1 tbsp.	15
Sauerkraut	½ cup	16
Seeds, pumpkin	1 oz.	13

Soy milk	1 cup	7
Soybeans	½ cup	16
Tomato sauce, spaghetti, marinara	½ cup	17

Vitamin K Free (less than 5 mcg)

Food	Serving
Bread and cereal products	1 oz, or ½ cup
Cheese, all types	1 oz.
Eggs	1 large
Fish and shellfish	3 oz.
Fruit, whole, canned or juice	1 each or ½ cup
Meat and poultry, all types	1 oz.
Milk and dairy products, all types1 cup	1 cup
Nuts, not previously listed	1 oz.
Seeds, sunflower	2 tbsp
Vegetables and vegetable juice not	
Previously listed	½ cup

Sources

1. U.S. Department of Agriculture, agricultural Research Service.2008 USDA National Nutrient Database for Standard Reference , Release 21. Nutrient Data Laboratory Home Page http://www.ars.usda.gov/ba/bhnrc/ndl__accessed October 2008.
2. Nutrition Data. Com: Nutrition Facts and Information , http://www.nutritiondata.com; accessed April 28 2008

Tips for good cooking

Over the course of time I have done a lot of experimenting with cooking following healthy diets. Some have turned out real good and some went straight into the trash can. The key is learning to work with what you can eat. Follow your doctor's guide lines for healthy eating.

We only go out once a week to eat and it is somewhere that has a healthy menu. If when you are dinning out and you have a question don't be afraid to ask what the contents is of what is on the menu.

I happen to love to cook so experimenting makes healthy eating being fun. There is no salt of any type in our house. We cook only with Mrs. Dash and pepper. Mrs. Dash has a lot of different spices and they can be combined to make great tasting dinners.

I like gravies but packaged gravies are high in sodium. I found a way to have good homemade gravies using Mrs. Dash. Once I put the meat in the pressure cooker I follow cooking instruction but I add ½ cup of water extra. I then add what flavors of Mrs. Dash into the pot and cook as the recipe calls for. If I want thinner style gravy I let the juices simmer a little longer. If I want thicker gravy I put a little in a frying pan then add 1 Tbsp. of flour and brown then add the rest of the juices to the consistency I what.

We do not fry any food; it is broiled, baked, boiled, or grilled. We also use a counter top grill that cooks on both sides at once.

What you can eat healthy is only limited by your imagination and creativity. I am eating better now than I ever have and plus I lost 40 pounds, and feel great.

Here are a couple recipes that I created that fits my dietary needs,

The first rule is follow your doctor's guidelines and be very vigilant about being complainant.

Uncooked Turnip Relish

This recipe for relish is for people that take Coumadin and like relish but can't have it because of the Vitamin K in cabbage. We replaced the cabbage with fresh turnip roots. It is very good as a condiment or as a side dish. This is a small batch so as not to worry about canning a large amount. It can be stored in the refrigerator.

Ingredients	Amount
Turnip root, med	3
Carrots	2
Onions, small	1
Bell Pepper, Green	½
Bell pepper, Red	½
Bell Pepper, Yellow	½
Vinegar	2 cups
Sugar, White	¼ cup
Mustard Seed	1 tbsp.
Celery Seed	1 tbsp.

Using a food processer grind up all vegetables, mix them together and let drain. After completely drained, mix all ingredients together except the vinegar. After mixing start pouring in the vinegar mixing slowly. Taste often and stop vinegar when you like the taste and consistency. Put relish into jars and store in the refrigerator.

Pizzas are high in sodium and made with processed meats. So we needed to come up with one that would fit into my dietary needs.

Ingredients

Corn tortilla

Ground turkey

Cheese, shredded, low sodium

Onions, chopped

Peppers, chopped

Tomatoes, diced

Spaghetti sauce, low sodium

Place Corn tortilla on pizza pan an spread 2 tbsp. of sauce over the tortilla. Brown the ground turkey and sprinkle all over the tortilla. Add all the other ingredients evenly over all the pizza. You leave off or add but look at the sodium content before you put it on the pizza. Place in oven at 400 degrees until cheese melts

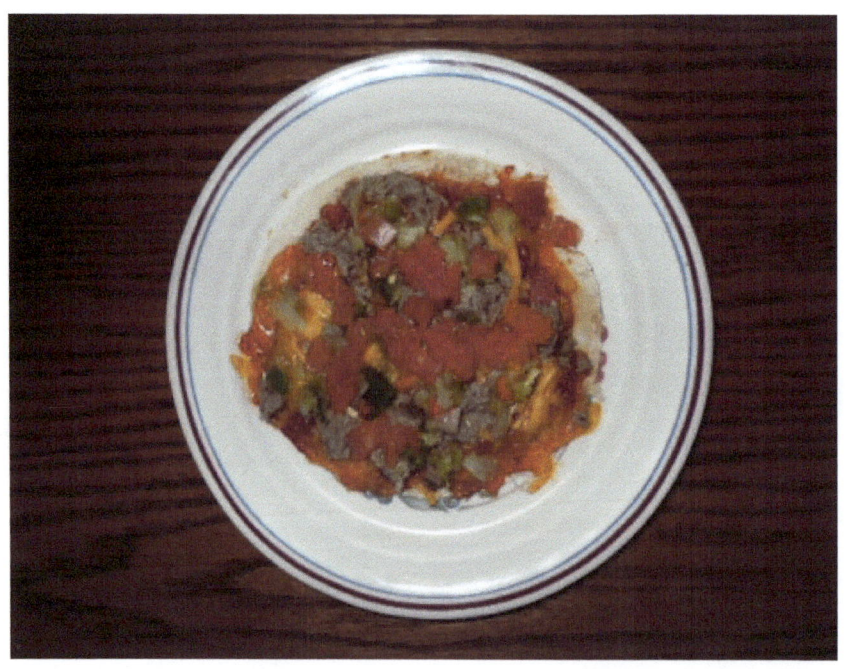

Low Vitamin K Salad

Being on Coumadin I need a very low Vitamin K diet. That takes salads off the menu, which I like a lot. Here is another recipe that I adapted too that works out very well for me. It is sort of a cross between a salad and slaw; you can adjust to your taste.

Ingredient	Amount
Bell Pepper green	¼
Bell Pepper red	¼
Celery stalks	3
Tomato, small	1
Onion	¼
Carrots, Baby	8
Cheese, low sodium	1 Tbsp.
Olive Oil	2 Tbsp.
Vinegar, Red malt	2 Tbsp.

In a food processer grind the Bell peppers up, they will make a lot of liquid, don't drain. Dice up the rest of the ingredients and mix them all together. Pour the Olive oil and Vinegar over the salad and then sprinkle shredded cheese over the salad.

Reflective Remarks

The key to living good after a major medical issue is Compliance. The doctors know what the best path to follow is. This does not mean you cannot get second opinions, but following the rules is a necessity. They can give you the guidelines but it is up to you to follow them. We all want to live a good healthy life but after the hospital it is up to you.

I have tried to provide some tips on buying and preparing good healthy dinners that are also a pleasure to eat. There are a lot of recipes that you can experiment with. Create your own to your taste and style. When you make new ones write down what you do and how you can change it the next time if you need to.

The charts in the back are what I used to follow my doctors guidelines and it worked rather well. It provided me a look at how close I was following the guidelines. You can also bring the charts to the doctors' visits to let them know what and how you are doing.

Sometimes I would think is it not worth it, but let me tell you "It Is Worth It". The doctors and staff are there to help you and they will help you in every way. All you have to do is ask and follow the guidelines.

Compliance is what makes all the difference

How to use the charts

The Following are examples of how to use the charts

Blood Sugar Checks

Used to track Blood sugars and weight

Date	Breakfast	Lunch	Dinner	Bedtime	Weight
3-10-14	117	120	101	110	192
3-11-14	105	118	110	125	192
3-12-14	109	120	118	124	193

Food Contents

Used for shopping purposes until you get use

To shopping with your dietary restrictions.

Item	Serving size	Sodium	Sugars	Cholesterol	Calories	Other
Brand Name	2/3 cup	0mg	4g	0mg	70	
Brand Name	¼ cup	80mg	25	15mg	200	
Brand Name	10 oz	5mg	5	8	45	

Sodium, Sugar, and Calorie Count

This chart is for tracking the intake of different contents at meals and snacks

Date	Sodium	Sugars	Calories	Vitamin-K
3-10-14 Breakfast	110mg	120g	350	40mcg
Lunch	211mg	25g	402	4mcg
Dinner	320mg	58g	625	57mcg
Snack	5mg	120g	425	74mcg
Total	646mg	323g	1802	175mcg

Examples Only

NOTES

Blood Sugar Charts

Date	Breakfast	Lunch	Dinner	Bedtime	Weight

Weight is taken before breakfast and blood sugar taken before meals

NOTES

Food Contents

Item	Serving size	Sodium	Sugars	Cholesterol	Calories	Other

NOTES

Sodium, Sugar, and Calorie count

Date	Sodium	Sugars	Calories	Vitamin K

NOTES

www.ingramcontent.com/pod-product-compliance
Lightning Source LLC
Chambersburg PA
CBHW060826290526
45792CB00005BB/1810